21 Forever with Makeup

Professional Makeup Tips & Advanced
Techniques That Make You Look
Stunningly Beautiful & Years Younger

Evelyn R. Scott
Copyright© 2014 by Evelyn R. Scott

21 Forever with Makeup

Copyright© 2014 Evelyn R. Scott
All Rights Reserved.

Warning: The unauthorized reproduction or distribution of this copyrighted work is illegal. No part of this book may be scanned, uploaded or distributed via internet or other means, electronic or print without the author's permission. Criminal copyright infringement without monetary gain is investigated by the FBI and is punishable by up to 5 years in federal prison and a fine of $250,000. (http://www.fbi.gov/ipr/). Please purchase only authorized electronic or print editions and do not participate in or encourage the electronic piracy of copyrighted material.

Publisher: Enlightened Publishing

ISBN-13: 978-1499538595

ISBN-10: 1499538596

Disclaimer

The Publisher has strived to be as accurate and complete as possible in the creation of this book. While all attempts have been made to verify information provided in this publication, the Publisher assumes no responsibility for errors, omissions, or contrary interpretation of the subject matter herein. Any perceived slights of specific persons, peoples, or organizations are unintentional.

This book is not intended for use as a source of legal, business, accounting or financial advice. All readers are advised to seek services of competent professionals in the legal, business, accounting, and finance fields.

The information in this book is not intended or implied to be a substitute for professional medical advice, diagnosis or treatment. All content contained in this book is for general information purposes only. Always consult your healthcare provider before carrying on any health program.

Table of Contents

Introduction 5

Chapter 1: Properly Prep for Better Makeup Application 9

    Clean your skin... 9

    How and when to cleanse............................ 12

    Exfoliate to help your makeup work better 16

    Moisturize for more even makeup 19

Chapter 2: Creating a Good Foundation 25

    Prepping with a primer............................... 25

    Clean up your complexion with concealers 27

    Applying concealer 29

    Setting your foundation 30

    Finish with powder...................................... 35

Chapter 3: Tricks with Highlights and Contours for a More Youthful Face................ 37

Make your nose appear smaller 39
Bring out your eyes 39
Define your cheeks 40

Chapter 4: Younger-looking Eyes 43

Age-appropriate eye makeup 43
Pairing eye color with shadows 46
The right way to use eye liner 48
Get great lashes 50
Define youthful eyebrows 54

Chapter 5: Glowing Cheeks 59

Types of blush – powder, creams, gels 61

Chapter 6: Age-defying Lips and Nails 67

Applying color 70
Choosing a lip color 72
How to apply the ultimate lip color 73
How to choose the best nail color 75

Chapter 7: Makeup that Lasts and Other Tips to Look Younger 77

Finish with powder 77
Secrets to long-lasting makeup 78

Makeup that older women should avoid . 81
Have the right tools 84
Know when to swap out makeup............... 87

Conclusion 91

Introduction

At a young age, we are introduced to the power of makeup. Used in the right way, makeup can transform pale eyelashes into alluring, flirty fringe ... or create a sensual pout on otherwise thin lips ... or create a glowing look for cheeks that are less-than vibrant.

We're told that the key to good makeup is to enhance our natural good looks and play up our best features. Judicious use of certain makeup is key to pulling this off. In the beginning, we use just a touch of lip gloss and a hint of eye color. But with experience, we become more experimental and play with bold colors on our eyes and get adventurous with wild nail polish. It's one of the many joys of being a girl and getting to play with pretty and playful colors.

As we age, of course, we tend to tone down the shades we use and want a more youthful look. While many women turn to expensive skin creams and surgical enhancements, those who care for their skin well can actually use makeup to create a younger-looking complexion. With a few tips and tricks and the right products and tools, you can master the skills needed to use makeup as a temporary fountain of youth.

You need to start with clean, healthy skin, so we've included tips in this report about how to create a great complexion that works as the canvas for your makeup. This is an important step that cannot be skipped.

For aging skin, we include many insider secrets that makeup artists know will make their clients look years younger, like properly exfoliating your skin and which type of cleanser will work best. From BB creams to concealers to highlighting and contouring, applying makeup is about much more than simply adding some color to your lips, eyes and cheeks. You can actually reduce the look of fine lines, make your cheekbones look higher, shrink a wide nose, shape your eyebrows to best frame your face and boost the volume of both your lashes and lips that may have thinned over the years.

And the best part is that you will not look like you've over-done your makeup application. It can still look natural while effectively concealing the years. You'll learn how to choose the right colors for your eyes, cheeks, lips and overall skin tone and you'll find out which products work best for your skin type. One you get your new routine down, people will notice that you look more vibrant and youthful, but they won't even be able to figure out why. So if you want to learn how to look like you're glowing from within, read on …

Chapter 1: Properly Prep for Better Makeup Application

Before you can even consider what type of foundation will give you the coverage you need, or which colors play up your eyes the best, you need to ensure that your face is well cleansed, moisturized and exfoliated. These steps will guarantee that your skin is free of clogged pores that can cause your makeup to look dull or caked on. What you're going for is makeup that looks natural, accents your best features and—best of all—helps to make you look years young. Here's where to start:

Clean your skin

While it may be refreshing to give your face a rinse with water, that alone won't do enough to clear out the pollutants, dead skin cells and makeup on your skin. If you don't remove those three factors, your complexion will look dull and your other beauty products—and especially your makeup—won't work as well on your skin. So if you're using an expensive serum or moisturizer, you're only getting part of the benefit if your skin is not fully cleansed.

As we age, our cleansing needs change because our skin becomes more fragile and can be easily damaged. You'll want to look for a cleanser that is labeled as "gentle"—or ask for help from a store professional before you purchase it. As a general rule, if a cleanser makes your face feel too tight afterwards, it may be striping away too much of your natural oils. Try to pair your cleanser to your skin type—most will say if they are best for dry, oily, sensitive, aging or combination skin. Here are some of the different types of cleansers you may want to look for and how they react to different skin types:

- **Gels**. A cleanser that is a gelatinous form will say "gel" on the label. This are good for people with oily skin that has frequent acne breakouts because gels typically don't leave much product behind once they are rinsed off.

- **Foams**. Foaming cleansers are typically gentler and wash away clean without drying your skin. They're ideal for normal skin types. If you have dry skin, avoid cleansers that include alcohol or sulfate. Some cleansers that are geared to acne-prone skin may have ingredients like salicylic acid in them—just check the label to ensure there are too many acids included, because they can irritate your skin.

- **Oils**. If you have dry skin and need to retain more moisture, an oil cleanser may be your best option. Plus, it will leave your skin feeling smooth.

- **Soaps**. A bar of soap is super convenient, but look for those that have natural ingredients like chamomile, tea tree and lavender oils. You'll want to choose a bar soap that is made especially for cleansing facial skin. Body soaps used on the face can cause excessive dryness.

- **Lotions or milks**. These are ideal for aging skin because they leave a slight moisturizing residue behind once they're rinsed off. Since aging skin may be dry on the surface, the extra hydration can be helpful.

How and when to cleanse

You may have been told that it's best to clean your face morning and night. However, if your skin is on the drier side, you might actually be doing more harm than good because it is removing the natural oils in your skin that help lock in moisture and keep your complexion looking bright and dewy. If you decide to go with a once-a-day cleanse, do it at night so you're not sleeping with a face full of makeup and pollutants that amassed during the day. In the morning, you can give yourself that splash of water to help wake you up.

To wash your face, pull your hair back and make sure your hands are clean, otherwise you'll simply get the grime on them on your face. Next, use a gentle makeup remover. These come in oil, liquid or cream form (like cold cream). You may want to experiment to see which you like best. Take care around your eyes to remove all makeup, but keep your eyes closed to avoid getting product in your eyes. Applying the makeup remover with a cotton ball will give you the best control and help you avoid getting any in your eyes.

Next, use warm water to give your face a splash and then to work your cleanser into a lather. Hot water may cause your capillaries to burst and cold water can tighten your pores too much. You may find that some of the newer cleansers on the market do not include foaming agents (which can irritate some skin), so they may not foam up very much. Using your fingertips, work the cleanser into your face with gentle, circular motions all around your face. Do not pull or be too harsh with your skin, as it can easily be damaged—no matter what your age.

Rinse well with a clean washcloth to ensure all of the cleanser is gone—or else your skin may get dry and feel tight and excess residue can attract dirt to your face. When drying your face, simply pat it with a clean towel and do not rub the towel into your face, as this can also cause damage, especially to skin that is warm and wet.

If you have oily skin, you may want to follow your cleansing routine with a toner, which is typically a watery liquid that helps to draw impurities out, remove what your cleanser may have missed and help to reduce the appearance of your pores. Some toners are soothing, with ingredients like chamomile. Others are astringents that include alcohol—avoid these if you have dry skin.

Others include exfoliating ingredients that can help to cleanse more oily skin. Other toners may simply refresh the skin, which is great for those with dry skin who only cleanse their skin at night. If you have dry skin, in the morning, splash your face with water and follow with a skin freshener.

In addition, if you work up a sweat or use heavy hair products, you may also want to consider adding a wash of your face during the day. Both can clog your pores and cause more bacteria to grow, which will inevitably lead to blemishes. If you notice pimples along your hairline, it's likely due to your hair products.

Once you've cleaned your skin, don't wait too long before you continue with your other skincare products, like serums and moisturizers. When your skin is warm and slightly wet still, it is in the optimal state to absorb these products more effectively. If you allow your face to fully dry, they may simply sit on the surface of your skin without soaking in. When you apply makeup on top of products that have not fully soaked into your skin, the makeup may not blend evenly around your face and can easily look caked-on and obvious, rather than glowing and natural.

At the end of the day, it's important to remove your makeup. Even if you're tired or don't feel like cleaning away the makeup on your face, it's an important step because if you leave your makeup on all night, it will have another eight hours or so to clog your pores along with the rest of your day's dirt and grime. Also, it will smear off onto your pillow, which makes for an ideal breeding ground for bacteria and dirt. Night after night, if you sleep on a dirty pillow, you're increasing your chances of developing an acne breakout.

Use a makeup remover with a cotton pad to remove your makeup. If you have oilier skin, follow up with your regular cleanser. If you have dry skin, you may not want to wash twice a day. Instead use a cleanser at night after you've removed your makeup, and simply use a toner before your moisturizer in the morning.

Exfoliate to help your makeup work better

You'll want to give your skin a bit more of a deeper clean by using an exfoliating product once or twice a week to fully remove dead skin cells that are clogging your pores. Those dead skin cells can make your skin look dull and create a perfect breeding ground for your skin's oil, dirt and lingering makeup to form pimples.

Exfoliating products come in many different forms and ingredients. The most common is the use of a scrubbing mechanism, such as salt, sugar, finely ground nuts or apricot seeds or other agents that are a bit abrasive. Sometimes synthetic "microbeads" are included to slough away any lingering impurities, makeup and dirt. They are typically blended with a cream and foaming agent to make it easier to smooth across your skin.

Some ingredients in beauty products that you can purchase over-the-counter and use daily also have exfoliating properties, like retinol or alpha hydroxy acids. Retinol is a vitamin-A derived exfoliant that also helps to strengthen your skin, fight acne, improve cell turnover in your skin and even reduce the signs of aging (like fine lines and wrinkles) as well as sun damage. If you buy it over the counter, look for "retinol." If you dermatologist thinks you need a stronger form of it, he or she will prescribe you "retinoids." It's an ideal, non-scrubbing exfoliant for aging skin, but use caution as it will make your skin more sensitive to the sunlight. Use a sunscreen every day to avoid getting a sunburn (which you should be doing whether you use retinol or not).

Alpha hydroxy acids are especially effective at cell rejuvenation, as they help to remove older skin cells to make room for fresh ones. It's believed that alpha hydroxy acids also help to boost collagen production under the skin. Collagen is a natural substance below the skin's surface that keeps skin looking plump and youthful. Collagen production slows as we age, so many beauty products are now geared toward helping speed it back up, and alpha hydroxy acid is a key ingredient.

If your skin needs a deeper clean, schedule a visit to the med-spa or the dermatologist office for a microdermabrasion treatment, which is a deeper scrub exfoliation, or a chemical peel that utilizes stronger forms of acid like glycolic or salicylic acids (among others) at prescription strengths. Chemical peels come at varying strengths and will cause the top layer of skin to eventually "peel" off after it has healed from being exposed to the acid. These are treatments you'll only need occasionally (perhaps once every month or two), but are excellent for improving the tone, texture and color of aging skin—all of which set a better base for your makeup and allow you to use less makeup since blemishes, pigmentation issues and fine lines and wrinkles may be dramatically reduced.

At-home Exfoliators

If you'd like to experiment with a scrubbing exfoliator, choose one that is labeled for your skin type. Using them in the shower is ideal, because the steam will help to open your pores. After cleansing your skin, take a small amount of the exfoliator (about a quarter-size drop) and rub it between your fingertips to activate the ingredients. Some exfoliators will even warm up a bit.

Next, gently rub the exfoliator into your skin in circular motions, similar to how you clean your face. Continue this soft massage for a minute or two all over your face and neck (avoiding your eye area). Rinse thoroughly and pat your face dry. You'll only need to use a scrubbing exfoliant once or twice a week. However, if you use beauty products that contain other exfoliating ingredients like retinol or alpha hydroxy acids, a scrubbing exfoliator may not be necessary and might even cause skin irritation. Also, do not use body exfoliation products on your face—they are far too abrasive.

Whatever form of exfoliation you choose, afterwards you will definitely notice that you need to use less of your skincare products and makeup. Plus, your makeup will smooth on easier and will be easier to blend, which is essential to getting a natural look. So don't skip this important step.

Moisturize for more even makeup

Now that your skin is free of pore-clogging dirt and grime, it's time to replenish some moisture, which is important to keep aging skin looking dewy and supple. Well-moisturized skin will also work better with the formulas of powdered makeup like eye shadow and blush.

When the skin's chemistry is out of synch, it can cause surface dryness that needs to be rehydrated. A moisturizer will help your skin hold on to hydration that might otherwise be lost to environmental factors, age or even a change in weather. They don't actually add water to the skin, but provide ingredients that help the skin retain it below the surface.

There are many different types of moisturizers, and choosing one for your skin type can be challenging. Those with oily or combination skin will want to stay away from oil-based formulas. However, these types should not skip moisturizer all together because aging skin needs the extra hydration. Dry-skin types can handle thicker cream moisturizers. Whichever type you choose, it should leave your skin feeling soft and smooth, but not greasy or as if there is a layer of the product "sitting" on your skin. (Following the cleansing and exfoliating steps outlined above can help your products to absorb more efficiently into your skin.)

After you've cleansed and used your toner, apply your moisturizer right away while your skin is still slightly damp. The moisturizer will lock-in that hydration all day. Pick a lighter-weight moisturizer for day use, and look for a thicker nighttime moisturizer to work while you sleep.

When choosing a facial moisturizer for aging skin, ingredients like alpha hydroxy acids, hyaluronic acid, ceramides, peptides and squalene as well as botanicals like vitamin C and E and even fatty acids that will nourish the skin in a deep and effective way.

However, you'll want to avoid some common ingredients like shea butter, wax, lanolin oil or mineral oil, as these are believed to cause breakouts, disrupt the production of your skin's natural oils and even lead to early wrinkles because they disrupt normal cellular activity. If you're in doubt, have your skin analyzed by your dermatologist to find out what type of moisturizer you need.

Double-duty Moisturizers

Luckily, many manufacturers are developing all-in-products, like moisturizers that have a light tint of color that are great for those who don't want to apply a heavy foundation. They can also provide a little bit of coverage for fine lines, blemishes and discoloration on your face. Plus, it makes getting out the door that much quicker and if you choose one just a shade darker than your skin tone, you can even achieve a light bronze self-tan without relying on the sun, which will damage your skin with repeated exposure.

That's why many moisturizers today also include sun protection, typically SPF 15 or 30. Because protection your skin from the sun is vital as you age, you'll want broad-spectrum SPF protection every day all throughout the year. The sun can cause dreaded age spots and actually saps moisture out of your skin. Some products offer all three in one bottle: moisturizer, tint and SPF. Some fear that one ingredient may outshine the others, but formulas are constantly being improved, such as the so-called "BB creams" that are new to the market.

BB creams originated in Korea as a way to combine multiple ingredients in one application and create a flawless finish. The term "BB" has various meanings—usually beauty balm or blemish balm—which make promises to fix any imperfections, like lines or pimples, while moisturizing and protecting the skin. It's a foundation, moisturizer, SPF, antioxidant and primer all-in-one. Since formulas vary widely, be sure to check the ingredients to get what you want (not all have SPF, for instance).

Experiment with different brands to find one that improves your skin's texture while providing much-need coverage and protection. Some are more opaque than others and some go on more smoothly, and you may still want your foundation beforehand if you have aging skin with surface dryness.

Chapter 2: Creating a Good Foundation

Getting creative with a variety of colors for your cheeks, eyes and lips is the fun part, but you have to start with an evenly toned complexion. There are a number of products that can help smooth out imperfections and create a blotch-free, pretty surface for your color palette.

Prepping with a primer

Before you begin applying makeup, you may want to start with a primer. These specially developed formulas are geared toward creating a smoother finish to your skin to set the canvas for your makeup. While your moisturizer may be at work hydrating your skin, any roughness, blemishes or unevenness can be addressed by using a primer.

Primers typically include silicone polymers for their filling abilities. The polymers can fill in lines, improve the appearance of pores, and improve the overall texture of the skin by fixing all of these minor flaws. By creating a smoother surface, a primer can also keep your makeup from sinking into fine lines or acne scars that can cause the makeup to look cakey, especially your foundation.

Primers can also eliminate shine and even eliminate that afternoon oiliness that can plague more oily skin. If that type of shine is an issue, you might opt for a powder primer, although you can also find primers in balms, lotions or gels. You can also find formulas for specific parts of your face, such as cheeks, lips and eyelids.

If you have oily skin and you're concerned about adding yet another layer of product on your face, look for a primer that's specifically geared toward preventing and even healing blemishes. Oily and sensitive skin types may also want to avoid the synthetic silicone polymers and look for a primer with botanical ingredients filled with natural antioxidants. They may not fill fine lines as well as the polymers, but you'll likely get some shine protection and a smoother surface.

Some primers are best used over your moisturizer and under your foundation, however, some can also be used over your makeup to set it and keep shine away. Be sure to read the instructions thoroughly before applying primer on top of makeup.

Clean up your complexion with concealers

We all have problem areas that need more coverage than the average foundation can resolve. Under-eye circles, blemishes, acne scars and fine lines may need a bit more product to smooth out your face's tone. Concealers are ideal products to do this, and there are many types to choose from.

Concealers are sold in stick or solid form as well as liquid or cream varieties. Stick concealers, which looks similar to a lipstick tube, are ideal for oily skin because they stick to the skin better. They may also be a better option for those who have not developed many fine lines yet, as the drier texture of a solid stick concealer may get cake-y and crease or crumble on skin with deep lines. Once you apply this type of concealer, use the pad of your ring finger to gently blend it into your skin.

Cream or liquids are ideal for light coverage that you can apply in thin layers. The thinner the formula, the lighter it goes on and the less you will use. Some cream concealers will also include anti-aging ingredients like peptides to help plump areas that need a little extra attention, such as the under-eyes.

While many concealers are skin-tone colored to blend seamlessly with your foundation, there are several pastel-colored options that do specific work. After applying these colored concealers, follow up with a concealer that matches your skin tone to perfect your skin.

- **Peach and pink**: If your under-eye circles have a blue or gray tint to them, a peach- or pink-colored concealer can help neutralize them. It's also better for olive or dark skin.

- **Green**: These will help neutralize any redness or blemishes on your face, such as acne, rosacea or birthmarks. It may also help to reduce the look of minor scars.

- **Yellow**: Redheads or those who have a pink undertone to their skin will benefit from yellow concealers.

- **Purple and blue**: If your skin has a yellowish tint to it, a blue- or purple-toned concealer can brighten it up.

Applying concealer

If you need more coverage, you'll want to apply concealer before your foundation. If you just need a little help, smooth it on after your foundation. Either way, be sure to thinly layer it on. You can experiment with layering it before, after or maybe even a thin layer of both to get extra coverage for a night out on the town. Either way, be sure to moisturize your skin so that the concealer blends well and doesn't flake off as the day or night goes by.

For the under-eye area, start by applying a small amount to the inner corner of your eyes and sweep it across the area under your eye, paying special attention to the outer corner of your eye as well. Do not use a tone of concealer that is too light, or you will have a "raccoon" type of look below your eyes that's obvious and unnatural.

For blemishes, pat a yellow-toned concealer to cover redness onto the area and gently blend it. You may need a little extra primer first so the concealer stays put. For areas of uneven coloring, use a thicker cream concealer to even the tone. Some liquid concealers have a wand with a sponge tip that makes it easier to get apply in certain crevices, such as the sides of the nose. Some concealers can also act as highlighters, which we'll discuss in the next chapter.

Setting your foundation

As many types of faces as there are, there seem to be just as many types of foundation. Thick, lightweight, powder, spray, foam, liquid, creams, balms … it's an almost overwhelming host of options. The texture of the foundation will depend on whether you want heavy coverage or just a thin layer. Creams and balms give thicker coverage while foams, lightweight liquids and even powder foundations give just a bit of coverage.

Plus, if you have oily skin, you may want to opt for an oil-free "mattifying" foundation—although if you go too matte, you skin can look chalky, so be sure to test it first. Foams that dry with a powder-like finish are a good option for oily or combination skin. Dry skin types may want a more moisturizing option with ingredients like hyaluronic acid, which helps the skin to retain moisture and also acts as an effective anti-aging agent. If your skin has a fairly even tone, you might opt for a tinted moisturizer, as discussed in chapter 1, to avoid getting too many layers of makeup on your skin, which can look cake-y and create an aged look to your face.

If your skin is sensitive, you may want to look into mineral foundations, which are free of synthetic ingredients, like preservatives, or fragrances. Instead, they incorporate things like titanium dioxide or zinc oxide. They naturally offer sun protection and won't usually lead to blemishes or irritate your skin the way some makeup can. They often include many botanicals and plant extracts that offer anti-aging effects and nourish the skin.

When purchasing a foundation, it's best to go to a store where you can test it first. Judging a foundation simply by looking at the jar or tube will not allow you a realistic idea of how it will look when slathered all over your face. Arrive at the store with a clean, moisturized face so that you can try different formulas without any makeup already on your face.

The salesperson will likely start by asking how much coverage you'd like, light, medium or heavy. Once you've determined the texture, next will be choosing the appropriate color. Select a few shades that seem close to your skin tone and sweep them across your clean cheek. Some people believe that using the inside of your wrist is best to gauge a color match, but to really find the best color, try it where you're going to actually use it—on your face.

The harsh fluorescent lights of a department store or a corner drug store can be deceiving, so take a mirror and look a the foundation shades in natural light (next to a window or outside). Check which color on your cheek seems to "disappear" into your skin. That's the one that best matches your natural skin tone.

Some foundations are simply creamy, while others offer a bit of illuminating shimmer. Go for creamy during the day and a little shimmer at night. The shimmery foundations can be a good option for aging skin, as they will capture light on the contours of your face and deflect attention away from the shadows of any wrinkles.

Many foundations offer additional ingredients with anti-aging effects and sun protection. If you have these ingredients in your other skincare products, such as your moisturizer, you don't need to double-up with your foundation. In fact, too many anti-aging ingredients can actually be irritating to your skin. Just as you wouldn't take a variety of medications with similar ingredients, you don't want to load up your skin—which absorbs the powerful ingredients.

To apply foundation, make sure any other makeup, foundation or medication you've applied to your face is completely dry. Use a very small amount of foundation and "dot" it around your face—across your forehead, on your nose, along your cheeks and on your chin. Remember: you can always layer on more makeup, but if you'll have to wash your face clean if you apply too much. Plus, too much foundation, layered with more makeup will simply make you look older.

You can use your fingertips to blend the makeup across your face, and the warmth of your skin may help it the makeup to blend. But you may get better, more even coverage with a makeup sponge or a foundation brush that allows you to get the makeup in hard-to-reach spots, such as the corners of your eyes are along the creases on the sides of your nose. Be sure to blend the foundation along your hairline and down your jaw and into your neck to avoid any harsh lines.

Using your fingertips will ensure that you're not wasting any foundation, which can be absorbed into a sponge or brush. While you may automatically wash your hands after applying foundation, you should also consider washing your sponge or brush. Brushes made specifically for applying foundation will absorb less of the makeup than a sponge will. Some makeup artists suggest adding a bit of water to a sponge to blend in a cream foundation more thoroughly.

Since they come into contact with your face, brushes and sponges can pick up the bacteria and oil, which will contaminate the sponge or brush. Repeatedly using these tools without cleaning them can encourage blemishes down the road. Use baby shampoo and water to clean them regularly.

Finish with powder

If you're happy with the overall look and tone of your foundation, you can "set" it with a light powdered primer, or opt for a powder. Powder does much of the same work that a primer does, but it is a finishing touch with some extra color. It can fix any imperfections with your foundation, lessen facial shine by absorbing excess oil, provide a matte finish and even help your makeup to last longer. As with most types of makeup, there are many options with powders, too.

If you don't need the coverage of a foundation, a powder can add just enough to finish your look at keep your skin from looking shiny. It's also a good option if you use a tinted moisturizer and want to finish up with a mattifying powder.

There are two general types of face powder: pressed powder or loose powder. Pressed powder comes in a compact, often with a sponge-like applicator, which is a good option if you want to take it with you and apply it on the road. A loose powder will give you a more natural look, but you'll need a large powder brush to apply it, and excess powder my float away from the brush, so applying just a small amount over a sink is best. A pressed powder in a compact, however, is best for quick touch-ups.

The color of your powder should match your skin tone, and simply leave you with a finished look. You shouldn't be able to see the powder sitting on the tiny hairs on your face. If you can, you've applied too much. Heavy powder can settle into any fine lines and accentuate wrinkles, making you look older than you are. Use a light hand with both foundation and powder, and you'll end up with an even, glowing, dewy complexion.

Chapter 3: Tricks with Highlights and Contours for a More Youthful Face

Your next step to creating a beautiful face is to apply highlights and contours that can actually highlight your best features and play down those you may not like as much. In fact, done correctly, you can even change the shape of your features with the use of certain makeup. You can make a nose appear small, define your cheek bones, play up your eyes and generally make your face look younger, more sophisticated and polished.

You'll use highlighting makeup to lighten certain areas of your face. This can be accomplished with a concealer that is a shade lighter than your skin tone or a cream or powder makeup that is specifically made to be used as a highlighter. Some have a slight shimmer to them, as the role of a highlight is to attract light, and with the shimmer, it works double-time. Highlights are typically white, nude or beige.

Highlighting areas of your face accentuates them and draws the eye to them and can even appear to "lift" them—especially the cheekbones or the brow bone, which both suffer from some sagging due to age.

Contouring makeup is used to darken strategic areas of your face. It can also be a concealer that is two to three shade darker than your skin tone or a darker foundation or a bronzer that is darker than your typical cheek color. Contours are typically tan, brown or even a deep, dark shade of red.

Contouring certain spots will help to make them look more chiseled and actually aid the highlighted areas to take more of the attention. Contouring can even help certain features look smaller, like a large forehead or wide nose.

When highlighting, it's typically best to apply the light shade to the center of your forehead, underneath the outside corner of your eyebrow, under you eye, along the top of your nose, the top of your cheekbones, in the center point of you lip (the cupid's bow) and on the end of your chin.

When contouring, apply the darker color to your hairline, typically at the temples, along the sides of your nose, the upper crease of your eye lid, below your cheekbones, along the jawline and even on the center of your neck.

Make your nose appear smaller

As we age, our noses tend to gain a bit more volume as the fat in our faces starts to droop down. The tip of your nose can actually appear much larger. You can combat that with a few highlighting and contouring tricks.

First, apply a small amount of highlighter down the center of your nose, which will bring attention to the top of your nose and your eyes. Use your contouring makeup along the full length of the sides of your nose, from tip to eyebrow. Blend the highlighter and contour color well. Finish with a light powder down the top of your nose.

Bring out your eyes

Small eyes, or eyes that appear to be sunken in, can be helped with some clever makeup techniques. Apply a neutral shade to your full eyelid. Then use the darker contouring color along the crease of the lid. You can also take that same color and use it as a soft liner under your lower lashes. Use the highlighter under the arch of your eyebrow and in the corner of your eyes to make your eyes appear bigger. Finish with a dark, glossy mascara for a complete look.

Keep in mind that well-groomed eyebrows can make a huge difference in how open and expressive your eyes are. All the makeup in the world cannot help if you have unruly, unkempt eyebrows that aren't shaped to help finish your look.

Define your cheeks

While there may be some other telltale signs related to aging, such as fine lines around the eyes or graying hair, it's a loss of volume in the face, particularly the cheeks that can really age your face. You lose facial fat and supportive collagen underneath the skin's surface, and that causes the cheeks to lose their plumpness, and eventually, as the facial fat moves down, it can create jowls along the jawbone that can really make you look older. But playing with high and low colors along the sides of your face can help restore the appearance of full, well-defined cheeks.

To accomplish that, start by applying a highlighter along the upper part of your cheeks below your eye and sweeping up toward your temple. If you suck your cheeks in, the hollows are where you'll want to apply your contour color. You should not go above your earlobe, nor should you go too close to the mouth or your face may end up looking too skinny. Blend the contouring color upwards slightly, and the highlight on the apples of your cheeks upward. Finish with your blush color to the apples of your cheeks and blend well.

Chapter 4: Younger-looking Eyes

Experimenting with eye color can be one of the most fun aspects of makeup application since you can get away with an array of colors that play up your eyes, match your outfit or just demand more attention. However, choosing the wrong colors or type of eye shadow can cause the wrong kind of attention.

Age-appropriate eye makeup

Unless you are a teenager, you should stay away from extremely bright eye shadow colors, such as turquoise or blue. Most blue shades of eye shadow also have a bit of metallic or glitter in them, which is another no-no for aging skin. Glitter can find its way into the crevices of fine lines and wrinkles and accentuate them in an unflattering way.

Also, using two tones of the same color (unless they are neutrals) can simply make your makeup look really heavy and dated. Any color on your eyes that goes too far from earthy or subtle colors is going to create a retro look that's not appealing and will make you look older than you are.

Another problem with glittery or unnatural color choices is that they will tend to crease more as the day goes on. Avoid these issues by trying the following steps:

- Use a primer on your clean lids that's going to help set your makeup and last all day.

- Use the darkest color in your palette to fill in the crease of your lid.

- Take some of a lighter color and blend the darker color in.

- Add some definition with a thin application of eye liner. The thicker the line, the smaller your eyes will appear.

If you'd like a bit more of a glamorous look without looking overly done, try these steps to create a smoky eye look:

- Choose a multi-toned eye shadow kit. They typically have three or four colors that have been pre-selected to work well together.

- After the primer and base color, add the lighter shimmery shade over your entire lid.

- Apply a darker shade over the crease and the outer corner of your eye that points toward your temples.

- Use the mid-range color to cover your lid and blend the lighter and darker shades a bit.

- Using a pencil or a dark shadow applied with a small contouring shadow brush to line below your lower lids.

- Use a pencil to line the inside rim above your lower lashes.

- Finish off with two or three coats of glossy black mascara.

So the basic application is a lighter lid, a dark crease and highlights under the brow and in the corners of your eyes. Keep in mind that you can always add more color in light layers, but if you've applied too much, it's difficult to remove it without simply starting over. You can play up your eyes with more liner and darker crease color, or go more natural with less liner. Whichever way you decide to go, be sure to use a generous amount of mascara to finish them off.

Pairing eye color with shadows

Generally speaking, you want to go with neutral colors on your eyes, and sometimes play them up with a surprising shade. Different eye colors look better with certain eye shadow colors. Here's how to choose one for your eyes:

- **Eye color for brown eyes**: Earthy shades of brown, bronze, beige and gold are ideal for creating big, soulful brown eyes. During the daytime, stick to champagne shades for your lighter lid color and soft browns for your crease. Sage greens are also a good pairing with browns. And pink can be a good all-over color that complements brown eyes well. For a bit of a surprise, try a dark violet in your crease or in an eyeliner. And while purple may be an unexpected choice, most skin tones can handle it.

- **Eye color for blue eyes**: Women with blue eyes already have a playful color to start with. To add more blue in shadow form would be a little over the top. Instead, go for more neutral shades like a light coral, gray, khaki or chocolate brown. A light, shimmery rose gold can be an ideal base color that easily blends with other shades. Blondes can get away with lighter shades and brunettes can go more dramatic with darker colors at night.

- **Eye color for hazel/green eyes**: Since many people with green or hazel eyes also often have fair skin, be careful in choosing colors that are too strong, as they will show up more on your fairer skin tone than they may on others. Opt for neutral taupe or light gold along with a bit of lavender to add a surprise element. If you have red hair, a brown shadow will really help your eyes to pop.

The right way to use eye liner

There's a lot of debate over whether using eye liner strategically enhances the look of your eyes or if the dark lining actually makes you look older. It can actually do both, especially with older eyes. If you are showing some signs of aging, and don't apply your eye liner correctly, it can look harsh and even accentuate fine lines and drooping lids. Here are some ways to use eye liner correctly to enhance the shape of your eye, rather than overwhelming it with too much color.

Unless you have dark skin and very dark eyes and want an overly dramatic look, you'll want to stay away from black eye liner. A better bet is to go for darker versions of colors that aren't quite black, like brown, grey, plumb or dark green. These shades look good with most eye color.

Different types of liner will create various styles of definition. A liquid liner will make a very distinct line that may be too harsh for aging eyes. A soft pencil liner can be blended a bit. And using an eye shadow with small, slightly wet eye shadow brush can create some definition that will help your eyes stand out and will blend well with the rest of your eye shadow color.

When experimenting with eye liner, start with the smallest line possible as close as you can get to your upper eyelashes. Blend it a bit so it doesn't look too severe. As with any makeup, you can always add more, but taking it off once it's on is a challenge. You may want to start with a pencil liner and follow with a darker shadow if you want more definition.

If you find that your eye liner starts to smudge during the day, try using some concealer close to your lower lashes and on your eyelid. Set it with a little powder, so that when you apply the eye liner, it's not sitting on bare skin. When your skin's natural oils secrete during the day, it can make any of your makeup run, which is why a good face powder is an essential element. Also, choose formulas that are waterproof and/or gel based to keep them from smudging throughout the day.

Something to keep in mind: If you are considering tattooing permanent makeup, such as eye liner or lip liner, onto your skin, think long and hard before you commit. No one truly knows what the cosmetic trends for the future may be, and "inking" on permanent liner may look really dated in a few years. And wearing dated, out-of-style makeup in shades that are no longer in favor is one of the surest ways to make you look older than you truly are.

Get great lashes

When you were younger, you probably had to use less mascara because your lashes were naturally think and long. With age, your lashes can think much in the same manner than your hair thins, due to stress, hormones or the natural aging process. The follicles that your lashes grow out of can become less efficient and you may end up with fewer lashes. Or those that you do have can be brittle and even breakable. You can pile on as much mascara as you want, but until you address your thinning lashes, you'll just end up with clumpy eyelashes that don't look natural.

Latisse is a prescription medication and the only eyelash growth drug that is approved for use in the United States. It works by extending the eyelash growth cycle, so that your eyelashes are growing for a longer period of time before they eventually shed, like any other hair on your body. Latisse is believed to play a role in lengthening, darkening and thickening the eyelashes. After using it for a few months, the vast majority of people see an improvement in one if not all of these areas. While it's been shown to be very effective, Latisse can cause your eyelids to darken and may even make your eye pigment turn brown. For those who have an adverse reaction, Latisse can cause redness, swelling and itchiness. Diligent and proper application can help to avoid issues like that.

Some over-the-counter lash enhancers don't help to grow more hair on your eyelashes, but they may nourish and protect the hairs you already have there, and keep them intact longer while new ones grow in. Many formulas include natural botanicals and peptides to do the trick. These enhancers may come with a mascara-type of brush to apply the enhancer all over your lashes. Others are simply a tiny brush that allows you to apply the enhancer right along your upper eyelids. If you feel discomfort on your eyelid, you may be putting too much on your lid.

One thing you can do to help keep your lashes looking lush is to be gentle with them, especially when using an eye makeup remover. Never tug on your eyes or your lashes or you could damage your skin and yank out lashes unintentionally.

Some hair-restoration physicians are experimenting with hair implants in the lashes, but because of the hair's curve, this type of surgery is difficult to achieve natural results, but they are getting closer to a solution all the time.

You can also create longer lashes with extensions that you glue in place (but these are difficult to maneuver) or you can have a professional apply a longer-term, yet still permanent, eyelash lengthener that sits on your lashes and adds length and volume.

The easiest way to add some length is by finishing your eye makeup with mascara. You may want to start, however, with an eyelash curler. Open the curler with your fingers and bring the device as close to your eye as possible. Clamp it down onto your eyelashes and hold for about 15 seconds. This will help the lashes curl upwards of the roots and allow your eyes to look more "awake," especially if you have rather straight lashes. Do not try to curl the tips of your lashes. This will result in a very unnatural curve of the eyelashes and can actually damage dry, brittle lashes.

There are many, many different types of mascaras on the market that promise to add length and glamour to your lashes, but you may need to try a few different versions to see which really work for you. They may include a typical round brush, or perhaps one that tapers at the end, or even one that looks like a tiny comb.

A round brush will add all-over coverage. A tapered wand will allow you to reach into the corners of your eyes where lashes are sometimes thinner, lighter and shorter. A comb-like want will help you separate clumped lashes that don't look good on anyone, no matter their age.

When applying mascara, take the wand and hold it right at the base of your upper lashes. Apply some mascara at the very bases of your lashes nearest to your eyelid. Gently move your wand against the lashes in a gentle, zig-zagging motion to really build up some product there. You can continue this zig-zag motion through to the ends of your lashes. Plus, it will keep your mascara from clumping. Let the first coat dry for a few minutes before adding a second coat. Apply mascara to your lower lashes by using the tip of the wand to carefully add color. Be sure to switch out your mascara every month or so, as it can collect bacteria and become thicker and clumpy.

Define youthful eyebrows

One of the mistakes that many women make is trying to drastically reshape their natural eyebrows because they want more of an angled brow, a thinner brow or a higher arch than their face can naturally handle. This is one of the quickest ways to age your face. Tweezing eyebrows too thin and coloring them in with a pencil creates an artificial, dated look that also makes you look older than you are.

Instead, enhance what you've got. There are some eyebrow shapes that you can build on to help to frame your entire face in a way that looks more balanced. You'll look more refreshed and pretty, and people who look at you won't even realize why. The first step is to determine the best shape for your face. Here's where to start:

For oval-shaped faces, which have a wider forehead that tapers to a thinner chin, a mostly straight eyebrow with a lifted arch that lines up just to the outer edge of your eye's iris.

Someone with a long face that doesn't taper as much as an oval-shape will benefit from eyebrows that are nearly straight across, with almost no arch. This will help to break up the balance of the face, so that it doesn't look so long.

A round face doesn't taper much to the chin, and is generally the same width bottom to top. This face shape can handle a more dramatic, angled arch that will actually make the face look less round.

A heart-shaped face can look very youthful, but the chin can sometimes be too pointy. Soften any sharp features by creating a rounded brow with a naturally curved brow.

A face that has a strong, square jaw can be easily balanced with a strong, angled or rounded eyebrow.

One of the most confusing aspects of creating great eyebrows is choosing the right color. They key is to play off your hair color—and not go too far astray. If you're a brunette, your brows should be a shade lighter than your hair. For lighter-haired women, the brow should be a shade darker than your hair so that your brows are an added accent that stands out a bit. If you've lost a bit of eyebrow hair due to age, find a brow pencil or powder that's the right shade and lightly follow the shape you want to fill in the missing hairs. Avoid using hair dye to change the color of your brows. The results are too unpredictable and you could end up with odd, orange-tinged brows.

To avoid mistakes on your own, go to a professional eyebrow waxer or threader to get your brows in shape once a month. Explain the shape you want and bring pictures if you find the brow of a celebrity that you like and who has the same face shape as yours. Between appointments, you'll just need to do a little maintenance when your brows start to grow back in.

When you're cleaning up your brows, remember that the inside edge of your brows should line up with the inner corner of your eyes. If you have wide-set eyes, you can bring the brows a little bit more, but only moderately. The space between your brows that is basically as wide as the bridge of your nose should be free of hair.

If you drew a straight line from the outside of your nose to the outside corner of your eye and beyond toward your temple, this is how long your eyebrow should be. If you tweeze away the tail, your face will not have a strong frame and will look oddly narrow at the temples. Use a pencil to softly elongate the look of your natural brow.

The arch of your brow, if you desire one, should occur above your iris or slightly to the outside of your iris. The more dramatic the shape of the arch, the more attention it will attract. Remember that high arches make the face look longer, while straight arches make the face look shorter.

Chapter 5: Glowing Cheeks

The cheeks are one of the most important elements of a youthful-looking face, which comes as a surprise to most people. With age, the skin loses its natural glow and the volume of the face starts to diminish as well. While we don't want fat on our body, it's actually an asset in the face because a little extra fat makes the cheeks stand a little taller, giving a rounder, younger look.

While certain skincare treatments or even injectable fillers can help to restore the glow and volume of your cheeks, your makeup can be quite effective in creating the illusion of fuller cheeks—and less expensive and painful.

The role of blush is two-fold. First, it's used to create a natural glow. It's important to choose the correct color of blush for your skin tone. The ideal color of blush is the color your cheeks naturally turn after you've gone for a run and the blood has rushed to your cheek area a bit. Using this natural color as a guideline with help you avoid cheek color that is too off-base for your skin tone. You can also match your blush to your natural lip color. Typically, a dusty rose color works for most skin tones.

As a rule of thumb, you want to go darker than you natural skin color. So if you are fair-skinned, a blush with a pink hue will likely work best. But if you're darker-skinned, you can choose darker rose colors for your cheeks. If you have a warm tone to your skin, lean toward coral colors. If you skin has blue undertones, go for the burgundy family of blush shades.

The second role of blush is to play up shape your cheeks. You want to use blush on the apples of your cheeks to make them more pronounced than the other areas of your face. Do not make a dramatic swipe across your cheek toward your temple. It can easily look harsh and is typically unnecessary—unless you're starring on Broadway and need theatrical makeup.

By simply adding a bit of color to the round apples will give the illusion of a youthful glow that's simple to achieve. When applying your brush, smile into the mirror to accentuate the roundest part of your cheek. Focus your blush application on that rounded area, fanning it out and upwards slightly so that it blends and looks natural. This creates a nice look if you still have a good amount of facial fat that hasn't diminished with age.

However, if you need to add the appearance of volume, use your highlighter and contouring shade strategically. Suck in your cheeks and apply a deep bronzer in the indented areas. Apply your regular blush to the apples of your cheeks and fan it up and outward to blend. Then use a light highlighter—maybe something with a bit of sparkle—on the very tops of your cheeks, just below your eye sockets. The bronzer will deflect attention away from the hollows of your cheeks while the highlighter draws the light and the eye to the top of your cheeks, making them look more lifted.

Types of blush – powder, creams, gels

The most common type of blush that women use is a powdered blush, which is a great option to create a light, matte look to the cheeks. However, there are several varieties of blush that are good for different uses and different skin types. Here's what you need to know to choose the best blush for your skin:

- **Powder blush**: A compact of powder blush is best for oily skin types because it does not add any sort of liquid agent to the skin. Plus, it's simple to get just a bit of color, or to layer on more for a more dramatic nighttime look. If you're new to applying makeup, powder blush is a good place to start.

    To use a powder blush, choose a medium-sized blush brush and swirl the tip of the brush into blush compact to pick up some color. Tap the edge of the brush to get rid of excess blush. Smile and lightly brush the blush onto the apples of your cheeks. It's best for the life of your brush to move the blush in one direction, rather than swiping it back and forth or in circles.

    If you need more color, add another light layer. Be sure to blend up your cheek bones just a bit. You do not want a harsh line of color trailing to your hairline. Some powder blushes come in loose powder—especially mineral makeup. You can use the same technique, just be judicious with the amount of loose powder blush you take up on the brush to avoid excess blush on your face. A fluffier brush may work better with loose powder makeup.

- **Cream blush**: If you have particularly dry skin, a cream blush can add a boost of moisturizing ingredients while also adding color. Most cream blushes come in a small pot container. To avoid contaminating the makeup with the bacteria on your fingers, use a cotton swab or a makeup applicator to extract some cream blush out of the pot.

  Place a few "dots" of cream blush on the apple of your cheeks and up your cheek bones toward your hairline. There will be a lot of dense color in a cream blush, so focus on the apples of your cheeks, and lessen the color as you go up your cheek. Lightly smooth the blush into your skin by gently tapping in a swirling motion. Don't pull your skin, as aging skin can easily be damaged. Use your ring finger to blend in the cream—it is your least callused finger. Plus, using your finger will warm the cream blush a bit, which will allow it to blend more naturally. The final look should be a soft, well-blended glow. If you need more color, add another light layer.

- **Gel or tint blush**: These types of blushes usually come in a tube and are fast-drying, making them good for people with oily or normal skin who just want a hint of color. They can also work well for aging skin that needs a bit of moisturizer and protection. Look for a gel or tint blush with an SPF. A gel blush can give you a light glow that doesn't look like makeup at all, if you apply it carefully. It also is the longest-lasting type of blush. When using a gel blush, be sure your skin is well-moisturized, as dry skin will cause the gel to get streaky. In fact, you can add a little moisturizer or your foundation to your gel blush to avoid an unnatural look. Since it is fast-drying, you have to work quickly with a gel or tint blush, but adding a bit of moisturizer or foundation to it will give you a bit more time to perfect the look.

Squeeze a tiny amount of the gel onto your finger and dot it along your cheek line as you would a cream blush. You can use your fingers to blend it in, or a makeup sponge or brush that will blend it well into your foundation (don't apply a gel over any powder makeup, or it won't blend well). Add another layer if you need more color. If you apply to much gel blush or it creates a streak or goes in the wrong direction, you can clean it up with a little bit of moisturizing lotion and try again. Wait for the gel blush to completely dry before finishing with a powder or other makeup.

For a very natural, glow-from-within look, try applying a cream, gel or tint blush before you apply your foundation. Plus, if you've gone a little heavy with the color, your foundation and finishing powder will tone it down.

A word about makeup brushes: Because they pick up and retain makeup as well as bacteria and oils from your skin, you need to clean them regularly—at least once a month. Soak them in a bowl of water and makeup remover or baby shampoo for a few minutes (don't use regular soap, which can be too harsh and damage the brush bristles). Brush them onto your hand until no more makeup is coming off of them. Fluff them back into shape and stand them up in a container while they dry. Before using them in makeup again, re-fluff the dry bristles until they've recaptured their original shape.

Chapter 6: Age-defying Lips and Nails

You can make quite a statement with your lips—along with your eyes, they attract the most attention when you meet someone new. According to recent studies, men are more attracted to women who wear red shades on their lips, but not every red shade works on every skin tone. Plus, if you're playing up your eyes with more makeup, you'll generally want to play down your lip color—or vise-versa. Meanwhile, aging lips can make wearing bold lip colors a challenge. Here are some tips to creating beautiful lips that are appropriate for your age, while still looking sexy and appealing.

Your lips will start to lose volume as young as your 30s, especially if you are in the sun a lot without protection or if you smoke. When you smoke, your lips constantly make a puckering motion, which encourages the development of tiny, vertical lines on your top lip that can be difficult to get rid of and will cause your lip color to bleed. Women are more likely to develop these lines because they have fewer sweat glands than men do, which may help men's lip lines to stay more naturally hydrated. Drying skin, which is also made worse by smoking, is the enemy of youthful, full lips.

You may also experience a thinning of your lips with age since your face—including your lips—is constantly losing fat and collagen, which are two factors that keep the lips looking full. Unprotected sun exposure is the most common culprit in fat and collagen loss in the lips. No matter which lip balms, glosses or sticks you use, always choose those that contain some form of SPF protection.

Before you apply color to your lips, take steps to get them in great shape. Like the rest of your face, you'll want to exfoliate and moisturize your lips to get the best look for your lip color. As you may notice after spending a lot of time in extreme temperatures—either hot or cold—the skin on your lips will react by drying out and chapping. Once the skin on your lips has healed, try a gentle exfoliation to remove the dry skin and reveal softer, smoother lips.

You can find some products at drug stores or department store makeup counters that are made specifically for exfoliating your lips. Or you can make an at-home lip exfoliator by mixing a bit of table sugar with olive oil or honey and gently rubbing it onto your lips. All of the ingredients are natural, so you won't have to worry if some gets into your mouth. The more you rub it in, the stronger the exfoliation. Rinse well. You can also put a bit of petroleum jelly onto a soft toothbrush and gently "brush" your lips with it. The jelly will help your lips to retain moisture. If your lips are a little dry, simply wiping them with a clean wash cloth may be all the exfoliation you need.

Follow up your exfoliation with a moisturizer. Look for a lip treatment that includes ingredients that are known to add a substantial amount of moisture to the skin, such as shea butter, vitamin E, beeswax, jojoba oil or olive oil. Your lips will instantly feel soothing relief. You can follow up with a balm that includes sunscreen.

Applying color

Your first step is to choose which type of product you want—a lipstick, gloss, balm, or stain? And within each of those are more options—matte, shine, metallic and more. Here's how to narrow down your choices.

A tube of lipstick is the most traditional form of lip color—and for good reason. It's designed in a specific angle to glide over your lips, giving you maximum color coverage. And since the color is denser than other types of lip color, the pigment in lipstick naturally provides more protection from the sun—although many brands include extra SPF in their formulas.

Lipstick comes in three main styles—matte, for long-lasting color that is not too shiny; creamy, which is great for hydrating dry lips; and shimmery shades that are slightly frosted to make your lips look bigger.

Lip glosses are very popular now and draw a lot of attention to the lips. They do not allow for complete opaque coverage the way a lipstick does, and some glosses contain ingredients that may even make your lips more susceptible to sun damage, so choose carefully. That being said, some do contain SPF protection.

Lip gloss is available in shiny formulas as well as creamy colors that provide a bit more color. Some also include metallic sparkles for a nighttime look that also plays with the light to create lips that appear larger. If you want the coverage of your lipstick with more shine, simply choose a sheer lip gloss to apply on top of your lipstick.

Newer to the market are lip stains. These are popular because they give all-day color to the lips, but they can be drying to the lips. One way to get long-lasting color is to use a stain under your lipstick color or gloss. You'll need to experiment because some formulas don't work well together and cause the stain color to streak.

Lip plumpers are another newer item to the market that temporarily boosts the volume of the lips with certain ingredients. Using cinnamon, menthol or caffeine in the formulas can instantly plump up the lips up a bit. It's actually a slight injury that the ingredients cause which results in the plumping effect. It's not a dangerous injury by any means, but too much use can dry out the lips and they may sting a bit. Opt for a formula that includes peptides as the plumping ingredients, which also help aging skin to retain moisture. Of course, injections with lip fillers will semi-permanently add volume to the lips, but it's painful and can easily be over-done and create a very unnatural-looking "duck" lip.

Choosing a lip color

Picking a color that is not suited for your skin tone or creates too much of an unnatural contrast is a sure way to create a dated look that ages you. You can go dramatic with your lips—you just need to know how to pick the right shade.

For the perfect daytime look, opt for a lip color shade that is up to two shades darker than your natural lip color. Plus the color on one of your lips to compare it to your other lip. It's a good idea to sample lip shades with very little other makeup on that will distract from the lip color. Typically speaking, if you are fair-skinned, go for shades that have a bit of peach in them. If you medium or olive skin, go for a bit of rose-colored shades. If your skin is dark, you can go for deep colors like burgundy or even shades with a bit of chocolate undertones.

Every woman should have a shade of red lip color that she can use on special occasions. And even though many believe that can't or shouldn't wear red, that's not the case. The same rules apply—lighter-skinned women should lean toward warmer tones of red, like cherry, salmon or coral. Darker-skinned women can lean toward reds with cooler, blue or violet undertones. You can get these shades of red in lipsticks, glosses or stains for your desired amount of color.

How to apply the ultimate lip color

Now that you've found the right color for your complexion, it's time to properly apply it for long-lasting color that makes your lips look fuller and won't smudge during the day.

Start with a primer that's made specifically for your lips. Like a face primer, it will smooth out your skin and can even fill in minor lines along the top of your lip. Lip primers are typically clear or nude, so don't worry about going outside the lines of your lips. They are typically sold in lipstick-like tubes or squeezable liquid tubes. A lip primer will help your color stay on longer and may create a more even canvas for darker colors or red lip shades. Look for a primer that's packed with other benefits, like sunscreen and anti-aging ingredients like antioxidants and vitamin A, C and E.

Next, use a lip liner that is closely matched to your lip color. You do not want to use a lip liner that is a different color or much darker than your shade of lipstick or gloss. Using a matching shade will help to keep the lipstick from spreading into the tiny vertical lines above your lip. Plus, it will help shape areas of your lips that may not be well defined. However, do not line outside your natural lip line. Darker lip liners look old-fashioned.

Use a lipstick to fill in the rest of your lips with color with the tube, or opt for a small lipstick brush for more precision while you apply. You do not have to go over the lip liner excessively. Be sure to apply an even amount of lipstick to your entire lips. Blot lightly with a tissue to remove any excess that could end up on your teeth or bleed outside your lip line.

You can no apply a very light dusting of face powder to set the color in place and add another thin layer of lipstick. Next, apply a shimmery gloss to the fullest part of your lower lip and the middle of your top lip to make your lips appear larger. To further accentuate the shape of your "cupid's bow" where the top of your top lip dips, place some highlighting makeup there to catch the light and make your lips shapelier.

How to choose the best nail color

The traditional rule of thumb is to match your nail color to your lip color, but modern makeup rules are more lenient. As long as your lip and nail colors don't totally clash, anything else goes. If you are older and have hands that look more aged, you may think that adding color will only accentuate the aged look. But actually, the opposite is true. Using a nude color will call attention to crepey skin or sunspots. Instead, choose a brighter color—or one that contrasts against your skin tone—to add some visual interest and detract against signs of aging.

Today's trends allow you to have more fun with your nail color than ever before. If you are older than 40, however, it's probably best to stay away from the wild trends like blue nail polish, crackle polish, flower art or other designs. However, you can go for bright oranges, pops of red or shades of lavender.

The same rules apply for nail polish as with lip color—if you're fair-skinned, stick with warmer colors with pink or peach undertones. Darker-skinned complexions can go to cooler shades with blue undertones. You can certainly play off your lipstick color to pair with your nail color, or you can choose a color that complements your clothing for the day. However, nail color is typically fueled by trends or time of year. We'll typically go with pastels during spring, bright colors during the summer, earthy tones in the fall and deeper jewel tones during the winter. You can wear all of these shades no matter your skin tone; you just need to stay in the right family of colors for your skin tone.

One thing to keep in mind: As you get older, keep your nails on the shorter side. Neat, slightly rounded nails look more youthful than unruly, long, witchy-looking nails. Plus, shorter nails are less-likely to chip or splinter, which aging nails are more known to do.

Chapter 7: Makeup that Lasts and Other Tips to Look Younger

No matter how beautiful your makeup application may be, if you don't take steps to make it last throughout the day, it can be a streaky, creased mess by the afternoon. Here are some insider tips on how to avoid that.

Finish with powder

Once you have completed your makeup (except your mascara and lips) it's time to set your makeup with a powder. It should be the same shade as your foundation and can either come in compact form or loose powder. Powder that is pressed into a compact, called "pressed powder" on the label, offers more coverage, while a loose powder will give you lighter coverage. Before you apply your powder, make sure that your foundation has dried completely. Then, use a big, fluffy brush to take up some pressed powder and tap off the excess. If you're using loose powder, tap a little bit into the jar's lid and use the large brush to take up some of the loose powder.

Use the brush to apply it all over your face and neck with soft, circular and downward motions, using the brush to reach crevices. The powder will help absorb a little bit of oil, give you a matte finish and help your makeup to last longer throughout the day. You can also put some of the loose powder in your hand and use a fingertip to apply it to any crevices you may have missed with the brush, or in areas you want a bit more coverage, such as sun spots or blemishes.

Secrets to long-lasting makeup

Don't over-apply powder, because it will end up looking overly matte and cakey. You can always carry a pressed powder in your handbag for light touch-ups later. However, if you are covering up skin that has gotten oilier throughout the day, applying powder may be the worst thing you can do. It will not smooth on gracefully and your brush or applicator will get clogged with oil from your skin. Instead, try blotting paper. These ultra-thin sheets of paper are made specifically to sop up oil off your face without interfering with the look of your makeup. You simply need to press the paper against your skin without rubbing and it will wick away the oil that's making your skin look shiny. If you feel you still need powder, be sure to use enough blotting paper to remove as much oil as possible.

Another trick is to swap out some of your regular makeup during the warmer months of the year. If you use a thicker foundation during the winter, opt for an oil-free sheer tint during the summer. You can even get away with a tinted moisturizer or a BB cream, which won't clog your pores and won't look cakey later in the day if you live somewhere that is especially humid.

If you find that your eye makeup becomes creased by mid-day or wears away completely, be sure to include your eyelids when you are applying your primer before your foundation. If you don't have a primer that's acceptable for your eyelids, a concealer will work, as well. Either will help to keep the color in place and the colors will be stronger—and you'll end up using less. If your eye makeup still creases, use the tip of a finger to smooth the makeup back out, then use a brush to add a bit of color back in, avoiding your eyelashes. You can add a new layer of eyeliner, too, for some added definition. Use liquid or gel liners for color that lasts all day. Pencil liners are easier to apply, but they are more apt to wear away as the day goes on.

For your cheeks, try a gel tint during the hotter months, as they have more pigment in them and are more likely to stay put. If you like powder blush, you can apply a little extra in the morning. It will fade a bit as the day goes on and you'll still have a great look by the afternoon.

You will likely have to apply your lip color more than once during the day, but if you use a primer and a little bit of foundation on your lips before your initial application early in the day, it will help it to last longer.

Applying all of your makeup in light layers will also help it to last longer. But one major key factor is to choose oil-free makeup during the hottest days of the year. When you use makeup that contains oil (which can be helpful for people with very dry skin) it can actually warm up too much and smear off your face as the day wears on.

Keep in mind that liquid, gel and cream makeup will typically last longer throughout the day because the pigment in them is more concentrated. If you want to do a touch up later in the day, blot away oil first and layer on a thin amount of makeup. You may find that your skin takes up the color more quickly when your skin is warm and a bit oily. Along with blotting, you may also want to give your face a light mist. Many brands have created face misters that will not interfere with your makeup, but will give you a refreshing boost on a hot day.

Makeup that older women should avoid

Makeup trends come and go, and we're all tempted to give them a try. However, some types of makeup will actually accentuate fine lines and make you look younger. Here are a few types of makeup that are best to avoid if you have more mature skin:

Sparkly eye shadow. Shades that have a metallic shimmer to them used in concentrated areas, such as your eyelids, will actually make aging skin look worse. The glitter plays in and around fine lines, making the shadows of the folds in your skin more pronounced. Instead, opt for matte shades in neutral colors, such as taupe, champagne and peach, which look good on most people.

While matte looks better on your eyes, it's not a good option for your lips. Lip stains may last longer, but they can look harsh on aging lips that aren't as smooth as younger lips. Instead, opt for lip shades that are just a shade or two darker than your natural lip color and apply the color, followed by a shiny gloss. Your lips will look years younger.

A dark smoky eye and bold red lips may popular, but you do not want to wear both together. Play up one or the other, or else you'll look completely overdone, which is a sure way to look older. If you have a smoky eye, use a more neutral lip. If you have a bold lip, keep eyeliner and eye color light and neutral.

Swap out dramatic black eyeliner for a more subtle shade of brown or brown-black. You do not want to forego eyeliner all together because it is essential in creating definition to your eyes which may look more set back as you age. Do not create hard lines or "cat" eyes. Apply liner near our lashes and softly blend them. (Be careful not to tug on the skin around your eyes. It is very delicate and can be easily damaged.)

Pay attention to your brows as well. Use a conservative color that is not far from your natural brow tone, but be sure to fill in any sparse areas. This extra step will help frame your face and bring an overall balanced look. Also, be sure to curl your lashes, which may have lost some of their shape with age. This step will make your eyes look more wide open.

Nude foundation and lips may be all the rage for cutting-edge looks, but a more youthful look has a bit of natural blush to it. Staying within your appropriate color palette, look for shades that have a bit more pink in them. You can use these colors on your lips and cheeks to brighten up skin that may be looking a bit dull.

If you are having your photograph taken or will be on video, do like the celebrities do and wear more makeup. You may even want to have a professional apply your makeup before the shoot so that you'll have all the right highlights and lowlights that will create a camera-ready look. In the photograph or video, your makeup is dulled a bit, so don't worry about over doing it.

Have the right tools

Another great tip is knowing which brushes are used for which makeup. So many people simply guess, but like any project, having the right tools make all the difference. Here's a quick list of makeup applicators and brushes that will help you create a more professional look:

First of all, a good rule of thumb is to remember that you get what you pay for. Inexpensive brushes often do not have soft, quality bristles that make applying makeup more effective. If you invest a little more on your brushes, you'll get more out of them and they'll last longer.

A *foundation brush* looks most like an acrylic paint brush, with bristles that are packed tightly together. If you add a little water to a foundation brush, it will make application easier and more even. Be sure to wash this brush after every use.

A *concealer brush* looks like a mini version of the foundation brush. It can help you pinpoint difficult-to-reach areas and help you apply your makeup with precision.

A *dual-fiber brush* looks similar to a stencil paintbrush, in that it is flat and round at the end of the bristles and the bristles themselves are usually two toned (black and white or tan and brown). It is especially helpful in blending cream makeups such as foundation or cream blushes.

A *powder brush* is big, fluffy and soft. Load this brush up with loose or pressed powder—or even your bronzer—and tap off the excess before applying a thin layer of the powder on your face.

A *fan brush* may be a better choice for loose powders, as it will pick up just the right amount of powder and evenly distribute it across your face. A fan brush is helpful when you need to remove excess powder on your face. The fan shape makes it ideal for blending up and out, concealing fine lines in the skin.

A *blusher brush* is a smaller version of the powder brush, but the bristles are shorter and more tightly bound. The ends of the bristles are cut into a round shape, which perfectly complements the apples of your cheeks, making blush application natural.

A *contour brush* is perfect for use with contouring colors or highlights. You may want one for each product, so they don't mix. This brush is smaller than a blush brush and rounded.

Eye shadow brushes come in two sizes, one for all-over color and one for blending. The larger one can also be used for highlighting underneath your brow. An angled eye shadow brush is tapered to allow you to expertly apply a darker shade to your crease, which will add dimension to your eye makeup and make your eyes look bigger.

Eyeliner brushes vary from a fine-point brush that looks like a tiny paintbrush. It's ideal for liquid liners when you want a very thin line. You can also find flat, angled eyeliner brushes that have more bristles and allow you to get the liner well-placed at the lash line. You can also use it to extend the color up the lid a bit or to create a smoky or cat eye.

You will want two brushes for your brows—one to apply brow shadow, which is slightly slanted with stiff bristles. You'll also want a spiral-type brush that looks like a mascara applicator. This will help you comb your eyebrows into shape.

Finally, a *lip brush* may come with firm, short bristles, or longer bristles. Experiment with which one you like best. A lip brush may be quite helpful when using bold colors, such as red, because it gives you more control of where the color goes than a lipstick tube may do.

Know when to swap out makeup

Even though you may have your tried-and-true favorites, you'll really need to consider throwing out makeup that you've had for too long. Old makeup will not apply appropriately, may look old-fashioned and will definitely accumulate bacteria from touching your skin every day for several months. This can cause breakouts or negative skin reactions. Here's when it's time to go makeup shopping:

One of the tell-tale signs that your makeup has gone bad is that it will have a strange odor to it. Some people describe it as smelling like gasoline. Also, if you have a medical condition, such as pink eye or other skin disorders, you may want to swap out all of your makeup and start fresh once you've recovered.

- **Foundation**. If you do not touch the opening of a foundation with your finger and opt for a sponge instead, your foundation can last up to a year. The same holds true for your moisturizer. Your finger will contaminate the product and you'll need to swap it out after about a year. Also, face creams will lose their effectiveness if exposed to the environment too much. This can lead to irritation for your skin. Also, keep in mind that sunscreens have a shelf life of about six months to a year. If you opt for a combination product that has sunscreen in it, it may need to be replaced more often. The same holds true for many anti-aging ingredients, especially antioxidant and natural ingredients. They can turn rancid more quickly than synthetic products. Check the smell and color and if it looks off, don't use it. Natural products contain fewer preservatives and are gentler to your skin; however, they simply don't last as long.

- **Powders, eye shadow and blush**. Because these do not contain any liquids or water, they can last up to a year or even more. However, if you see that it has changed color or gotten wet, it's time to swap it out.

- **Pencil eye and lip liners**. These can last up to three years and should be sharpened regularly to expose new color.

- **Lipstick**. One way to keep your lipstick longer is to wipe the end of it with a tissue after each use. This will keep bacteria from breaking it down. Otherwise, replace lipstick every six months.

- **Mascara**. This is one of the worst culprits to accumulate bacteria. Be sure to swap out your mascara every two to three months, if not more.

- **Nail polish**. Look at the polish in the bottle and see if it has started to separate, which it will do anywhere from six months to a year.

Keep all of your makeup in a cool, dry place. The bathroom may not be the best area since it can get humid after a steamy shower. Wash your brushes every two to three months and wash your makeup sponges every week and toss them every month.

Conclusion

Now that you've mastered techniques to using makeup to create a more youthful look, you can start to experiment with other ingredients and colors to play up certain features. You may opt for different formulas for just about every type of makeup. Manufacturers are constantly creating new applicators for lip gloss and mascaras and there are often new ingredients added to our makeup that promise to give multiple benefits.

One of your best resources can be the makeup artists at department store cosmetic counters or other cosmetic stores. They are the experts of the newest and most advanced ingredient formulas. Most of the time, if you are simply in the market for a new product, the makeup artist will show you how to use the newer products in exchange for your purchase—and no other fee. Others will charge a small fee to do your makeup, which is a great way to experiment with new colors or brands without having to invest in the product itself.

Remember that applying makeup is one of the fun parts of being a woman where you can be playful, classic, chic or natural. Your makeup should enhance your good looks, and even improve them when you know how to use them correctly.

Made in the USA
Middletown, DE
11 December 2016